Living with Asthma

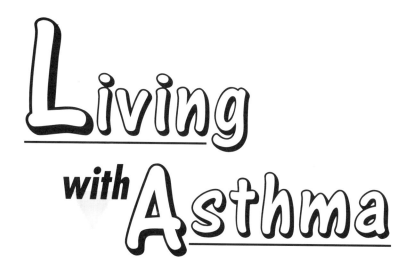

Living with Asthma

Margaret O. Hyde **and**

Elizabeth H. Forsyth, M.D.

Walker & Company
New York

The information in this book is not intended to be a substitute for ongoing care by a physician. Always ask your doctor about your own asthma control and management.

The people mentioned in this book are real, but in most cases their names have been changed to protect their privacy.

First published in the United States of America in 1995 by
Walker Publishing Company, Inc.;
first paperback edition published in 2000

Published simultaneously in Canada by Fitzhenry and Whiteside,
Markham, Ontario L3R 4T8

Library of Congress Cataloging-in-Publication Data
Hyde, Margaret O. (Margaret Oldroyd).
Living with asthma / Margaret O. Hyde and Elizabeth H. Forsyth.
p.   cm.
Includes bibliographical references and index.
ISBN 0-8027-8286-8 (hbk.).—ISBN 0-8027-8287-6 (reinf.)
1. Asthma in children—Juvenile literature.   I. Forsyth,
Elizabeth Held.   II. Title.
RJ436.A8H93   1995
362.1'9892238—dc20   94-41884
CIP
AC
ISBN 0-8027-7585-3 (paperback)

Book design by Susan Hood

Printed in the United States of America

2 4 6 8 10 9 7 5 3 1

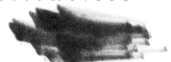

To Benjamin Williams Hyde

Contents

Acknowledgments

The authors wish to thank the many people who have contributed to this book. Dawn Sonn, R.N., Rachel, David, Kristin, Elizabeth, Emily, and many other kids with asthma were especially helpful. Thanks to the American Lung Association, National Jewish Center for Immunology and Respiratory Medicine, National Allergy and Asthma Network, and National Institute of Allergy and Infectious Diseases. Thanks also to the American Lung Association of Northern Virginia and the Fisons Corporation for supplying photos.

1

Does Someone You Know Have Asthma?

SOME kids who have asthma don't know they have it. Perhaps the most well-known symptom is *wheezing:* labored breathing accompanied by a whistling sound. Other common symptoms are coughing, shortness of breath, and chest tightness. But not everyone with asthma has all these symptoms, and not everyone with these symptoms has asthma. There are thirty-four other possible causes for wheezing. No wonder it takes a doctor to decide if a person has asthma.

More than 4 million kids in the United States under the age of eighteen do have asthma. One of them is Molly's ten-year-old friend Emily. Molly says that some of her friends think Emily has a terrible disease, while others think it is not any worse than having hay fever. Emily knows that asthma can be serious, but she has hers under control.

Molly had never thought much about asthma,

until Emily told her she had to avoid certain things or she would have trouble breathing. Emily looked perfectly healthy. She was a member of her school's swim team and the best diver in the school.

When Molly invited Emily and eight other friends to a sleepout in her backyard—to celebrate their graduation from fifth grade—the occasion brought home some of the problems that can trouble kids with asthma.

At first Emily was not sure she could attend the sleepout, because she had an *allergy* to some of the plants in Molly's garden. These plants made her eyes itch, her nose run, and caused fits of sneezing. When Molly's mother heard about Emily's problem with the plants, she carefully dug them out. So Emily could go to the sleepout after all.

At the sleepout, the girls talked more than they slept. One girl came late and brought an old sleeping bag that had been in the cellar. One girl complained that it smelled like mold, but Emily was asleep and did not hear the remark. Before long, Emily woke up with a tightening in her chest, gasping for breath, and coughing. She used her *inhaler* (a device that delivers asthma medicine in a vaporized form that can be breathed in), and soon her breathing returned to normal. The girl with the mold on her sleeping bag put it outside the tent and shared a big sleeping bag with another girl.

The next morning, all the girls were interested in Emily's asthma. She wished they would stop talking

Check Your

Asthma
"I.Q."

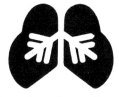

National Asthma Education Program

Prepared by the National Heart, Lung, and Blood Institute

The following true-or-false statements test what you know about asthma.

	True	False
1. Asthma is a common disease among children and adults in the United States.	☐	☐
2. Asthma is an emotional or psychological illness.	☐	☐
3. The way that parents raise their children can cause asthma.	☐	☐
4. Asthma episodes may cause breathing problems, but these episodes are not really harmful or dangerous.	☐	☐
5. Asthma episodes usually occur suddenly without warning.	☐	☐
6. Many different things can bring on an asthma episode.	☐	☐
7. Asthma cannot be cured, but it can be controlled.	☐	☐
8. There are different types of medicine to control asthma.	☐	☐
9. People with asthma have no way to monitor how well their lungs are functioning.	☐	☐
10. Both children and adults can have asthma.	☐	☐
11. Tobacco smoke can make an asthma episode worse.	☐	☐
12. People with asthma should not exercise.	☐	☐

1. True 2. False 3. False 4. False 5. False 6. True 7. True 8. True 9. False 10. True 11. True 12. False

about it. Feeling like you're strangling is bad enough without people making a fuss about it. Emily insisted that having asthma was not so bad if you followed a treatment program from a doctor.

Emily knows that she is just one of millions of people who have asthma. It is a great problem for some of them but just a time-consuming nuisance for others.

Lynette has asthma. She is a pretty seventeen-year-old who gets good grades and is on the bike racing team. She has had asthma for the last four years. She inhales medicine before races; it keeps her asthma under control.

Boyd has asthma, too. He is five years old and is ready to start kindergarten. He has had asthma for two years. His mother will tell his teacher about his asthma. She hopes that Boyd will not feel uncomfortable about using his inhaler in front of other kids in the class. Many young children with asthma are so used to caring for themselves that they take using their inhalers for granted. When a teacher explains at the beginning of the school year what the inhaler does, other kids in the class are not surprised when they see it. Boyd hopes that will be the case in his class.

Tricia, who is now a great-grandmother, says she has had asthma throughout her life, or at least for as long as she can remember. She is ninety-four. Some years the asthma was especially bad, but other years it did not bother her at all.

Forty-year-old Michael is not sure whether he has asthma. He has trouble breathing sometimes, but he thinks it may be because he is overweight. He says that everyone is short of breath after exercise, but he thinks he feels much worse than other people. He has been talking to friends who have asthma. They advise him to make an appointment to see his doctor to find out why he has attacks in which he is so short of breath.

Every case of asthma is different. It can be mild or severe. Newborn babies can have asthma, children can develop it at any age, and so can adults. There are more than seventeen million people in the United States with asthma, or about 5 to 10 percent of the total population! The number of reported cases rose 66 percent between 1982 and 1995. This may be partly due to more thorough and accurate reporting. No one really knows for sure. Asthma is the leading reason for children being admitted to hospitals and for being absent from school.

Asthma is the only chronic medical disease, other than AIDS and tuberculosis, that is on the rise throughout the world. Your chance of having or developing asthma is relatively small, but there is a good chance that you will meet someone with asthma at some time in your life. And that person will probably look as healthy as anyone else.

2

What Is Asthma?

ELEVEN-YEAR-OLD David was tired of continually answering questions from his classmates about his asthma. ("What does it feel like when your asthma is bad?" was probably the most common question.) So he asked several of his friends who had asthma to help with a program at their fitness club that would give others an idea what it was like to have asthma. A few of them said they would rather listen than be on the panel, but twelve-year-olds Ben and Rachel said they would join him. All three had suffered severe symptoms when they were younger, but now they had their asthma under control and all three of them were good athletes.

The panel knew the first question would be "How does it feel when you have asthma?"

David volunteered to answer it. He explained that when you have asthma, you have it all the time.

But there are times when you have an asthma attack—known as a *flare*—and then your "feelings" depend partly on how long the flare lasts, whether or not you know what is happening, and whether or not you have the proper medication. Some kids describe asthma as having "witches in my chest," feeling strangled, being in a state of terror, and expecting to die.

David asked everyone at the meeting in the gym to try an experiment that would help them get a sense of what it feels like when asthma flares. He passed out straws. Then he suggested that everyone stand up and run in place for two minutes. When he signaled the end of two minutes, they were to pinch their noses and place the straws in their mouths. Breathing with their noses pinched and the straws in their mouths gave them a rough idea of what it's like to have an asthma flare.

Most of the kids stopped pinching their noses soon after they reached this part of the experiment. David explained that people with asthma are not so lucky when they have trouble getting enough air to and from their lungs.

David then asked the kids how they felt when they could not get enough air through the straw. They described their feelings as scared, panicky, helpless, and awful. David said this is the way he feels when his lungs are screaming for air. At first, he was also embarrassed when the flares occurred at school, but now he knows that others are just anxious, and want to help him.

Even though people with asthma cannot suddenly stop gasping for breath, proper medical treatment can usually help them avoid these terrifying breathing problems. Taking medicine as prescribed by the doctor, avoiding triggers, and watching out for danger signs are ways of staying out of trouble.

The second question was "What happens to make people with asthma gasp for breath?" Ben set about answering this question with the aid of a chart. He stated that four problems cause the trouble in breathing: constriction of the airways, swelling, *inflammation* (invasion of white blood cells and fluid into the walls of the airway), and too much *mucus.* Then he launched into a detailed explanation.

The oxygen that you breathe is needed by all the living cells in your body. The blood that carries it to them is loaded up with oxygen in your lungs. The air you breathe goes into your windpipe *(trachea),* which you can feel at the front of your throat. This tube, which is made of a tough, rubbery material, goes down to the bottom of your rib cage. There it branches left and right into two tubes *(bronchi)* that carry the air almost sideways to your lungs. These two short tubes enter the lungs and then branch out about twenty-three times into *bronchioles,* almost like many twigs on an upside-down

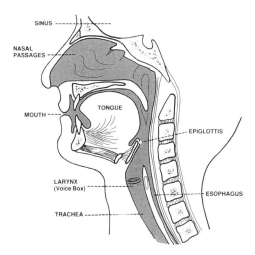

This cross-section of the head and neck shows the passages through which air gets to the lungs.

tree. The bronchioles open into small air sacs called *alveoli,* which are like tiny bunches of grapes but too small to see without a microscope. One hundred fifty million to 300 million alveoli are present. If they were spread out flat, they would cover an area almost the size of a tennis court.

Alveoli are amazing. Within the tiny walls of these delicate sacs are tiny blood vessels. The oxygen from the air you breathe is taken from the alveoli through the walls into the blood. The oxygen-rich blood is then carried to other parts of the body.

Carbon dioxide, a waste product, is also carried in the blood. It is released into the alveoli in much the same way that the oxygen came in. When you exhale, the used air, which contains carbon dioxide, is transported out of your lungs. It's a good thing you don't have to think about all of this when you breathe.

The tubes that carry oxygen and carbon dioxide have smooth muscles wrapped around them that can contract to narrow the tubes and restrict the flow of air. You cannot control these muscles, whereas you can control other muscles, such as those in your arms and legs.

The entire respiratory or breathing tree is lined with a special kind of moist, smooth skin called mucous membrane. Certain cells under the lining of the airways secrete a slippery substance called mucus, which protects the lining cells from infection and allows air to flow smoothly. When you have a cold, you blow a lot of mucus out of your nose. However, normally only about a tablespoon of mucus a day is produced in your respiratory tract. The lining cells of the airways have tiny hair-like arms that stick up into the mucus and move it along like a conveyor belt, carrying it up the airways, keeping them clear.

In people with asthma, the airways are supersensitive and tend to overreact. (This tendency is sometimes referred to as twitchiness.) In each asthma attack, or flare, the muscles wrapped around the air tubes contract, squeezing them and making them narrower. Then there is less room for air to flow through. At the same time, the linings of the airways become inflamed and swollen, mak-

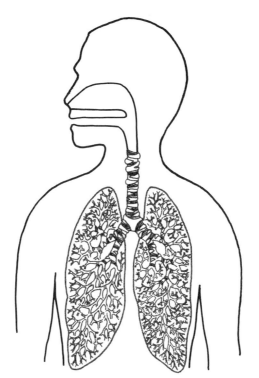

The air passages, or bronchi, branch like an upside-down tree as they get deeper into the lung.

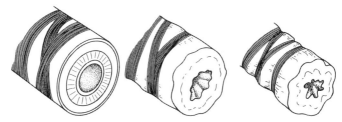

When the muscles that wrap the airways come in contact with smoke, dust, or anything else that acts as an irritant, they clamp down on the airway to keep the irritant from getting farther into the lung.

ing it even more difficult for air to flow. This causes the wheezing that is often heard in people with asthma. During asthma flares, a lot of thick mucus is produced. This mucus, in addition to white blood cells and cells that have been shed from the lining of the airways, sometimes form plugs that block the small airways. The persistent cough that is a symptom of asthma is the result of trying to bring up the mucus during a flare.

Breathing is a two-way street, with air flowing in and out of your airways at different times. The problem in asthma is not with breathing in but with breathing out. When there is an asthma flare, there is a traffic jam in which used air cannot get out of the lungs, so not enough fresh air can get in.

If you want to know how that feels, try the following: Take a breath, but don't breathe out. Then breathe in and out. Using the top of your lungs is very uncomfortable and tiring.

When all this happens, the person with asthma obviously has trouble breathing. He or she breathes more rapidly to try to get more air through the blocked airways. The ribs pull in. The heart races. If the case is severe, the person perspires. He or she cannot speak a whole sentence without gasping for breath after every few words. The skin may turn a bluish color (from lack of oxygen). If a severe attack is not halted, the person can die. Although the number of deaths from asthma is increasing, they are still relatively rare.

Rachel easily answered the third question: "Is asthma contagious?" She simply said, "No."

Next Rachel answered a question about how long an asthma attack lasts. She explained that asthma symptoms usually begin gradually and that they can get worse for several hours or several days. But sometimes symptoms are severe right away. When a person's asthma symptoms do not respond to medication, he or she is taken to the emergency room of the local hospital.

David volunteered to answer the question "How old are people when they get asthma?" This question had no specific answer. David said his doctor told him that it could start at any age, from newborns to the elderly. Most asthma attacks begin before the age of five or after the age of forty-five.

The final question was an important one: "How many Americans have asthma, and who are they?"

David told the kids that at least twelve million Americans have asthma. In children, asthma is more common among boys than girls, but in adults, it is more common among women than men. Asthma deaths are more common among African-Americans who live in poor urban areas, than among people who live in suburban and rural areas. No one knows why, but it may be partly due to living conditions and lack of access to health care in urban areas with large numbers of minorities and poor.

At the end of the meeting, everyone in the fitness group applauded the three members who had helped them understand more about asthma. Spreading accurate information on this subject is indeed a valuable service, for as we'll see in the next chapter, myths about asthma are in wide circulation.

3

Myths About Asthma

ALTHOUGH asthma is a very common disease and the number of cases has increased enormously in the last decade, many people still have wrong ideas about it. Some of these myths can do harm. Here are ten of the most common ones.

MYTH 1: Children outgrow asthma, so there is no sense in wasting money on doctors. Kids can just "tough it out."

This is both true and false. About half of the kids who develop asthma between the ages of two and ten will outgrow it. But it may come back later in life. Even if flares don't happen very often or don't seem serious, everyone with asthma symptoms needs to be under a doctor's care. Untreated asthma can keep kids from participating in games and sports with their friends. It can result in poor grades at school because of absence due to illness.

MYTH 2: Asthma does not need medical treatment.

People with asthma need medicine of some kind, even if their attacks are mild and not very frequent. (For details on medicines, see chapter 7.)

MYTH 3: Asthma does not kill anymore.

Asthma does kill people. About 5,000 people in the United States die from this disease each year. And the death rate has increased in recent years. Most people who die from asthma have not had enough help in controlling it in order to prevent attacks from becoming fatal. (We'll follow a near-fatal asthma emergency in chapter 4.)

MYTH 4: Smoking does not affect asthma.

Smoke is very irritating to the airways and is one of the triggers, or conditions, that sets off an asthma flare. (Triggers are the subject of chapter 5.) People with asthma should not smoke and should not be exposed to secondhand smoke. Kids whose parents smoke have a much higher risk of developing asthma.

MYTH 5: Asthma can lead to *emphysema.*

Other than in two extremely unusual conditions, a rare inborn deficiency of an enzyme, known as alpha-1-antitrypsin deficiency, and a rare lung infection called allergic bronchopulmonary aspergillosis, asthma does not lead to emphysema. Emphysema is most often caused by smoking. Emphysema is an irreversible disease in which the air sacs of the lungs are permanently damaged or destroyed. This interferes with the exchange of oxygen and carbon dioxide and causes shortness of breath. Asthma, on the other hand, is a reversible condition that affects the breathing tubes. People who have had asthma all their lives do not show any more damage in their lungs after they die than those who have never had asthma.

MYTH 6: Kids with asthma should not exercise.

Long ago, many doctors used to say that people with asthma should not participate in sports because it would increase their problems. Today, kids with asthma are encouraged to exercise. Kids and young adults with asthma have competed in every sport at a world-class level. Eight percent of the athletes who represented the United States in the 1988 Olympics had exercise-induced asthma. They were able to compete because they had proper treatment to prevent attacks caused by exercise. (See chapter 9 for a detailed discussion of asthma and exercise.)

MYTH 7: Moving to a different climate will cure asthma.

Some people with asthma feel better after they move from a damp, cold climate to a dry part of the country. But many individuals who pack their belongings and leave their friends and jobs to live in the Arizona desert are disappointed with the results. Usually, they discover that they are sensitive to new triggers that set off their flares. There is no guarantee that asthma will improve in a different climate. For those who are considering a move, experts suggest visiting the new place in all four seasons of the year.

MYTH 8: Asthma is all in your head.

Years ago, there was a widespread belief that children who developed asthma were born with certain psychological problems that caused their physical illness. We now know that asthma is a physical disorder that is not caused by the way you think or feel. Unfortunately, too many people still believe that asthma is "all in the mind." They think that kids with asthma can somehow control their wheezing and coughing if they really want to. Many physical conditions can be made worse by stress or things that are upsetting. Strong feelings like anger or even laughter can trigger a flare, but they are not the cause of asthma.

It is not hard to understand why kids with asthma sometimes get angry about their illness. They may resent taking medicine and always having to be careful about things that other kids don't have to worry about. Their illness makes them feel angry; the angry feelings do not cause the illness.

MYTH 9: Asthma is caused by a poor relationship between parents and children.

Jeff's asthma began when he was a baby. He seemed to be allergic to everything and had frequent flares that sometimes led to visits to the emergency room. His parents worried all the time. They did not allow him to play catch with his friends or ride a bicycle. They never let him go to summer camp or even to sleep at a friend's house overnight. They were afraid to leave him with a baby-sitter. By the time he was eight years old, he was convinced that he was a sick, helpless person who needed a lot of care and attention from everyone.

Then Jeff's father got a new job, and the family moved to another city. They found a doctor who helped the family deal with Jeff's asthma in a better way. He gave them a written plan that explained all about his medicines. Everyone close to Jeff learned more about triggers, how to avoid flares, and what to do in an emergency. The doctor suggested that Jeff's mother and father join a support group for parents of kids with asthma, where they could discuss problems and learn more about controlling asthma. They all began to feel more relaxed and confident. Jeff took more responsibility and stopped relying on his mother to remind him to take his medicines and use his inhaler. His mother let him join a swim club and allowed him to try other sports. Jeff learned that he was not really so sick and helpless after all.

Jeff's parents did not cause his asthma. But some experts once held mothers responsible; they wrote a book with the title *A Mother Originated Disease: Asthma.* These experts blamed the mothers of kids with asthma for sometimes being overprotective and other times not being attentive enough. It is true that mothers are concerned about their children's health, but this is a natural concern. It is also true that many parents, like Jeff's, are overprotective because they are worried. But the overprotectiveness is not the cause of the asthma.

MYTH 10: If someone in your family has asthma, sooner or later you may have it, too.

Although asthma tends to run in families, not everyone in a family will develop it. Scientists are learning more about the connection between asthma and heredity, but they have much to learn.

If you have asthma, believing these myths can be dangerous to your health. Misinformation prevents people from getting the care they need and can sometimes lead to an asthma emergency.

4

Asthma Emergency

ALTHOUGH kids who follow the doctor's instructions rarely die from asthma, asthma can kill. Let's follow what happens when a little girl named Marta has a life-threatening asthma attack.

Marta's parents call 911, and the sirens from the ambulance can soon be heard blocks away from the family's house. Her parents are glad to hear the sirens, for it means that their five-year-old daughter will soon be transported to the helicopter pad from which she will be flown to the hospital.

Marta lives on an island where there is no doctor. She has had asthma since she was born, and her mother and father have been told by all their friends that she would grow out of it. Her asthma was not severe before. In the past when she had an attack, her parents seemed to be able to help her breathe by holding her upright and fanning the air in front of her. She would wheeze for a while, but in a few minutes her breathing would be normal again.

This time was different. The coughing and wheezing did not stop. For a while, Marta was wheezing so loudly, her parents could hear her struggling for breath across the room. She was breathing rapidly, and the skin on her chest sucked in between her ribs with every breath.

At last the ambulance arrives. Marta's wheezing has stopped, but the medics say that this is an even more serious condition. There is not enough air passing in and out of her airways to cause the wheezing sound. A medic immediately gives Marta a quick-acting, inhaled medication to open her airways. He gives orders for the driver to get her and

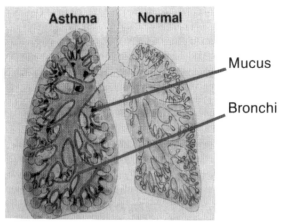

In this diagram, you can see how mucus clogs the bronchi of people with asthma. Compare the lung at left with the healthy lung at right.

her parents to the heliport as fast as possible. The medical team puts plastic tubing in Marta's nostrils; the tubing supplies extra oxygen from a container at her side. Another medic injects a needle into a vein in her arm. The needle is connected to plastic tubing that goes to a bag holding a solution of salt and water. The solution flows through the tubing and needle into Marta's bloodstream. She is probably dehydrated from breathing so rapidly, and this will replenish the fluid her body needs. The fluid will also help make the mucus thinner and easier to cough up. The intravenous line also enables doctors to inject other medicines quickly into her bloodstream if they need to.

When the ambulance reaches the heliport, the helicopter is ready. It lifts them into the air almost at once, and in ten minutes it lands on the roof of the hospital.

At the landing pad, the medics run beneath the helicopter rotors. They quickly pull the stretcher from the helicopter, put it on a gurney, a cart with wheels, and rush it into the building and into the emergency room. The medication has made Marta's breathing easier, but she still needs treatment. She may still have a dangerously low concentration of oxygen and too much carbon dioxide in her blood.

Marta is taken to the children's ward where she stays for several days so that the doctor can do tests and decide what medicines she needs. Marta's parents stay in the room with her. Before they leave, Marta's doctor assures them that her asthma can be controlled if they follow the directions he gives them. Their help in following the instructions is very important.

Marta's parents know much more about asthma than they did before her emergency. Now, they know that asthma can kill. They will never tell anyone that asthma is nothing to be concerned about. Although some children do outgrow this disease, many do not. It is important to follow a pattern of treatment to prevent emergencies of the kind Marta had.

Marta nearly died from asthma. As noted earlier, about 5,000 people die from this disease each year in the United States. This need not be. Dr. Michael Kaliner, chief of the allergy section of the National Institute of Allergy and Infectious Diseases, says that if the condition were properly treated, very few asthmatics would die.

Many young people are still suffocating from an entirely treatable disease. Asthma is not serious if medication is used properly, the way a doctor says it should be. But some of the medications for asthma work so well that users are lulled into a false sense of security.

This is what happened to an athlete named Mike Ivey, who had had asthma since he was eleven years old. Mike, a twenty-year-old, attended Catholic University in Washington, D.C., where he played football. He began using his inhaler much more frequently in the two weeks before he was rushed to the hospital, gasping for air. At the hospital, all attempts to help him failed. He died from asthma.

When Mike Ivey's lungs were examined after his death, a doctor remarked that she did not see how he could have breathed as long as he did. His airways were so inflamed, swollen, and clogged with mucus that he was getting almost no oxygen. When he used the inhaler, it opened the airways enough for him to continue temporarily, but it did nothing to heal the inflammation in his airways. He should have been using medicine for the inflammation. Needing to use the inhaler more often should have been a warning sign for him.

Most kids with asthma use their inhalers properly, but many children who have not been taught the proper steps to take in a bad attack, use their inhalers too often. Many inner-city kids do not have doctors who regularly care for them. They must depend on the help they get in an emergency room, and they tend to overdose themselves when an attack begins.

Inhalers are an important part of the treatment programs for kids with asthma. Such programs typically include avoiding the triggers that set off asthma attacks (see chapter 5) and taking medicine through an inhaler, by mouth, and/or by injection (see chapter 7). Unfortunately, some doctors do

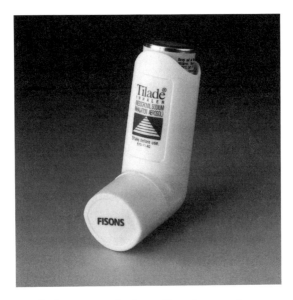

Inhalers are important tools for getting to your lungs some drugs that decrease inflammation and others that open the airways. (Courtesy of Fisons Corporation)

not put enough stress on the importance of the proper use of inhalers.

Asthma symptoms that do not respond to a person's usual asthma medicines are life-threatening. When this happens, a person suffers from what is called *status asthmaticus.* Typical reasons for severe attacks are: forgetting to take the correct dosage of medicine, not calling the doctor early enough, ignoring the fact that breathing is getting worse, and having a serious reaction to aspirin or other drugs. Aspirin, and products that contain it, such as Empirin, Ecotrin, and Bufferin, can trigger asthma attacks in some people.

A written medical plan to follow when normal medical treatment is not working has helped those who find themselves in an asthma emergency. If you have asthma, it is very important to seek medical attention at a doctor's office or hospital emergency room when you are not responding to your usual treatment. Ask your doctor to help you make an asthma action plan for emergencies. Ask her or him which emergency room nearest you is equipped to deal with life-threatening asthma.

5

Triggers

WHAT triggers, or sets off, an asthma attack? To answer this question, let's look at the experiences of several kids who have asthma, starting with two-year-old Sally.

Sally became sick with what the doctor said was the flu. She seemed to get better after about a week; her fever went away, and her nose wasn't so stuffed up. She looked healthy, but she continued to cough for months. The cough kept her awake at night, and the humidifier in her bedroom did not help. The doctor prescribed cough syrup, and some other medicine that he said would open the air passages, but nothing really made Sally better. The doctor said it might be a lung irritation from the infection, or perhaps an allergy to the family's dog. Her mother gave the dog away, but Sally still did not improve.

One night, Sally had a particularly bad bout of

coughing. She was having so much trouble breathing that her mother thought she might die. The family doctor was away, so Sally's mother took her to the hospital emergency room. After the doctor there heard her story and examined her carefully, he said he thought Sally had asthma. No one had ever mentioned the word *asthma* before, so Sally's mother was shocked. Despite her shock, Sally's mother was relieved. She knew that asthma is an illness that can be controlled by proper treatment.

Most but not all asthma sufferers wheeze. In some young children, like Sally, the illness may show itself as many colds during the year or even bouts of pneumonia (infection in the lungs), tightness in the chest, and shortness of breath. They may feel perfectly well with no breathing problems at all in between periods of illness. Without the wheezing, asthma is something that doctors do not always immediately suspect.

Years ago, doctors thought that children younger than twelve months could not get the narrowing of the airways that causes asthma symptoms. But, as mentioned earlier, asthma can appear at any age. More than half the cases start before the age of two.

In Sally's case, each bout of asthma was triggered by an infection caused by a *virus,* the tiniest of organisms. This kind of infection is the most common trigger of asthma in very young children and babies. Certain viruses, such as the flu virus, can act as triggers because they increase the twitchiness of the airways.

Colds and sinus infections (sinusitis) are very common triggers of asthma. If you have mucus dripping down the back of your throat, headache or pressure over your cheeks or forehead, and yellowish or greenish discharge of mucus from your nose, you may have a sinus infection. Treating the sinusitis is important in helping to control asthma symptoms. Viral diseases, such as colds, cannot be cured by antibiotics, but infections caused by *bacteria*—microscopic one-celled organisms—can be. (Strep throat is an example of a bacterial infection.)

It is difficult to avoid viral diseases, and no one would suggest that if you have asthma, you should be kept from school or from contact with other people. But it does make sense to avoid close contact with people who are sick with viral infections. And check with your doctor to see if you should get influenza (flu) vaccinations.

Other triggers of asthma are airborne substances that are inhaled into the lungs. Asthma is not an allergy, and not everyone with asthma is allergic. However, allergy is the number one cause of asthma. About 90 percent of children under ten years of age who have asthma also have allergies. Pollen from trees and plants (like ragweed), molds (which grow in damp areas both inside and outside the home), animals, feathers, and house dust are some of the most common substances that cause allergic reactions.

Dan learned that he had asthma when he was thirteen years old. He could deal with the inconvenience of it all, but how could he part with his cat?

When he was tested to find out what triggered his asthma, he found out that cat *dander* was high on the list. (Dander is like dandruff, or tiny scales that are shed from the skin and hair.) Since Dan's cat had long hair, his friends thought he might get along better with a cat with short hair. But it is not the hair that causes his problem. Cats of any kind are likely to be a problem for people with allergies.

About six million people in the United States are allergic to cats, although not all of them have asthma. Cats produce a protein that is made in certain glands in their skin. This protein coats the cat's fur, and when the cat licks itself to take a bath, it gets into the cat's saliva. When particles of the saliva get into the air and are inhaled they trigger asthma in some people.

Dan read that washing a cat with water at body temperature might help get rid of the cat dander. When he learned that someone would have to wash the cat for ten to fifteen minutes many times, and that the decrease in dander might take three to eight months, he decided to give his cat to a friend and get a snake or tropical fish. Dogs are less likely to be a problem for people with asthma than cats are, but Dan did not want to get attached to a dog and then find out that he had to part with it.

Twelve-year-old Jennifer wondered why she always developed a stuffy nose and sneezed and coughed most of the night when she slept over at Beverly's house. She never had any problems like that at home, until her mother replaced the old synthetic-filled bed pillows with new pillows that were filled with down feathers. Then they realized that Jennifer was allergic to down, and after a visit to an allergy specialist for tests, their suspicions were confirmed.

You do not get an allergic reaction the first time you are exposed to an allergy-causing substance. Your body needs a period of time before it becomes sensitive to that substance and reacts to it. For instance, Jennifer did not have any reaction to feathers the first few times she slept at her friend's house.

Throughout your body tissues, especially in the mucous membranes, are special cells called *mast cells.* After a period of exposure to an *allergen,* or allergy-producing substance, your body produces *antibodies* to that substance. In an allergic person, the antibodies that are produced stick to the mast cells and cause them to release chemicals that act on the mucous membranes, producing the runny nose, itchy eyes, and sneezing. These chemicals can also trigger an asthma flare. This is what happened to Jennifer. The same reaction occurs in people who have hay fever or who are allergic to other substances like house dust.

House dust is made up of many different kinds of tiny particles that float around in the air. Mold spores, bacteria, insect parts, and dander from humans and animals are a few examples of these particles.

The most common cause of allergy to house dust is a creature that is less than one-tenth the size of a grain of sand. It is the dust mite, whose scientific name means skin eater in Greek. Dust mites live in clothing, drapes, furniture cushions, and bedding, all places where flakes of human skin are plentiful. Your bed probably contains two million mites. Mites themselves do not cause any harm or diseases, but their droppings floating around in the air cause problems in people with house-mite allergy.

Other irritating substances like polluted air, paint fumes, car exhaust, burning leaves, perfume, and deodorants can also cause asthma flares. As noted earlier, one important trigger for asthma is cigarette smoke. Parents should know that if they smoke, their children have a greatly increased risk of developing asthma. Children with asthma have as many as 70 percent more flares and wheeze longer when there is a smoker in the house than those who are not exposed to secondhand smoke. There is no doubt that cigarette smoke is harmful to people with asthma.

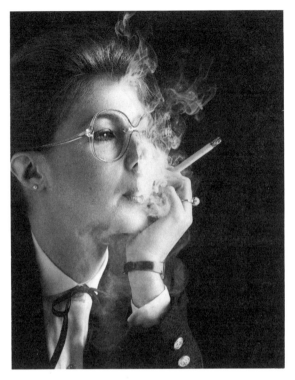

Cigarette smoke is a common trigger for asthma. (Courtesy of the American Lung Association)

Some children have food allergies that trigger asthma flares, but this is not very common. They are much more likely to be allergic to aspirin or other painkilling drugs, like Motrin. Some of the latter reactions can be severe.

Chemicals added to foods and medicines can trigger attacks. The greatest offenders are the chemicals known as *sulfites*. Sulfites are added to many foods, including dried fruits, molasses, beer, wine, and wine vinegar in order to keep them fresh. About a million people with asthma are sensitive to sulfites, and many develop very severe reactions if they eat or drink substances containing large amounts of sulfites. The Food and Drug Administration requires labels on any product that contains sulfites and bans the use of sulfites on fresh fruits and vegetables served at salad bars.

Jon is typical of about 80 percent of kids with asthma. For them, strenuous exercise is the trigger. Unlike flares caused by viral infections, exercise-induced asthma symptoms usually disappear about two hours after they begin if the person's airways were functioning normally before the exercise. Jon's asthma started in junior high school, but it did not stop him from participating in soccer, baseball, and basketball. He never missed a game because of an asthma attack. He is now a senior in college and is on the varsity tennis team. He takes medicine by mouth daily and uses an inhaler regularly. He has learned that before every game he needs to inhale additional medication to prevent a flare of his exercise-induced asthma. If he did not do this, he would experience wheezing and chest tightness in the middle of a game. Jon considers his pregame treatment part of his warm-up, like stretching.

Some asthma experts think that strenuous exercise triggers asthma because it lowers the temperature of the bronchioles. During exercise, cold, dry air is breathed in rapidly without having had a chance to become warmed and humidified in the nose and upper airway. For this reason, swimming is less likely to trigger a flare than other sports, since the swimmer is breathing humid air. Running, especially in the winter, and cross-country skiing are much more likely to cause asthma symptoms because they expose the person to both triggers of exercise and cold air. Many runners, ice-skaters, and skiers overcome these obstacles by using medicine and by wearing masks or scarves over their faces to protect against the cold. (See chapter 9 for more details on asthma and exercise.)

Fred is a twelve-year-old with asthma that is usually under control. Sometimes he has asthma attacks triggered by cold, and during hay fever season they are triggered by his allergy to ragweed. He is rather high-strung and sometimes flies off the handle, especially during a heated argument. At such times, he is likely to start wheezing. Does this mean that his asthma is caused by psychological problems? Not at all. Shouting, crying, and laughing can stimulate a nerve that causes the bronchioles to narrow, which in turn causes wheezing. If he were in a play and had to act angry and shout, he would probably start to wheeze, even though he was not really feeling angry. Although asthma is not caused by psychological problems, it can be made worse by stress or tension.

*I*f you have asthma, do you know which of the items on the following list triggers your flares? You may be sensitive to some things that are not on the list, but here are a number of the common triggers:

Infections such as colds or sinusitis
Allergies
   Pollen
   Mold
   Animals
   Feathers
   House dust
Irritants in the air
   Smog
   Perfume
   Cigarette smoke
Foods
Sulfites
Aspirin or other medicine
Exercise
Cold air
Shouting, crying, or even hearty laughter

Now that we've covered the common triggers of asthma attacks, let's consider in more detail the steps kids with asthma can take to avoid them. Some of these triggers are more easily avoided than others. For example, if you have asthma and no one in your house is a smoker, you don't have to worry about secondhand smoke triggering a flare. If you live in an area where the air is clean and free of pollutants from factories, then smog is not a problem. On the other hand, if you live in a smog-filled area, this may be a case where moving to avoid asthma flares is a sensible solution.

You may be allergic to aspirin, or sulfites, or to certain foods. Although giving up a favorite food may not be easy, it is probably better than risking a severe asthma attack.

Suppose you find out that you are allergic to your dog or cat. It is very difficult to give up a pet that is like a family member, but sometimes it is necessary. Like Dan, you may decide to get a snake or tropical fish instead. If you cannot give up your cat or dog, perhaps it could live outdoors. If it can't live outside, the next best solution is not to allow it in your bedroom.

What if you are allergic to house dust? As mentioned earlier, the big offender is the dust mite. The numbers of dust mites can be reduced by treating carpets with a chemical mite killer and using a special kind of vacuum cleaner that does not blow particles back into the air, as ordinary vacuums do. Mattresses, springs, and pillows should be covered with plastic casings. Bedding should be washed in hot water. Since mites live wherever dust collects, it is important to get rid of as many dust-collecting items as possible. Bare floors that can be mopped are better than carpeting. Shades are preferable to

drapes or curtains. Knickknacks and stuffed animals are dust collectors, too. Special air filters can
be installed in your house to help keep the air
cleaner. Forced hot-air heating systems blow dust
around, but filters placed over grates can reduce
dust.

Some asthma attacks are triggered by an allergy
to molds. Molds grow in places where there is a lot
of moisture—in damp basements and around bath-
room fixtures, for example. Sometimes molds also
grow in humidifiers or vaporizers, so these should
not be used in homes where someone is allergic to
mold. If a house is damp, a dehumidifier should be
used to dry the air. Outside the house, mold may
also be found growing in piles of dead leaves and
in mulch and compost piles. Ruth is allergic to
mold, so she does other chores while her mother
rakes the leaves in the backyard.

If you are allergic to pollen, there is not too
much you can do about avoiding the air outside.
Using air-conditioning in your house and keeping
your bedroom windows closed at night during the
pollen season can help. Running car air condition-
ers will also cut down your contact with allergy-
causing pollen that might otherwise blow in
through open car windows.

What about getting allergy shots? Are they the
best way to ward off such problems? Not necessar-
ily. Doctors do not give as many allergy shots today
as they did in the past because not everyone needs

them. They now know that only kids who have specific allergies that trigger their asthma should get shots—and only if the allergic substance cannot be avoided and if medicine does not work.

Consider the case of fifteen-year-old Maria. She dreaded the fall, even though she loved to hike in the mountains and enjoy the beautiful colors of the leaves. She always experienced severe asthma flares that did not occur at other times of the year and which could not be controlled completely by medicine. She went to an allergy specialist for skin tests and found out that she was allergic to ragweed pollen. The doctor started her on a series of shots. Maria has been taking the shots regularly for several years, and she has hardly any symptoms of hay fever. Her asthma is under control, and she can again enjoy the fall.

Sometimes, no specific cause or trigger can be found for a person's asthma flares. Even though there is no cure for asthma, and the triggers cannot always be avoided, there are many excellent drugs available to control it. These drugs are a great improvement over earlier treatments for asthma.

6

Old-time Treatments

LONG before today's medicines for asthma were discovered, doctors and parents tried a wide variety of substances and techniques to help children and adults with asthma. Many of these treatments seem harsh or strange to us now, but they were not viewed that way at the time. Consider, for example, the asthma remedies used by three famous individuals.

Marcel Proust (1871–1922) developed asthma when he was nine years old, and he continued to suffer from it in later years. In spite of his asthma, he was able to write novels that are considered some of the best of the twentieth century. He tried some odd remedies for his asthma—one of his favorites was drinking cold beer. Unfortunately, he did not take good care of his health and died at the age of fifty-one.

If you are interested in dance, you may have

heard of Robert Joffrey (1930–1988) or the Joffrey Ballet. Robert Joffrey began dancing after a doctor suggested it might help to control his asthma. At the time such a prescription seemed very strange since the benefits of exercise in controlling asthma were as yet unknown. Joffrey died in 1988 from a liver problem that was believed to have been caused by medicine he was taking for his asthma.

Theodore Roosevelt (1858–1919), who was president of the United States from 1901 to 1909, was subjected to many strange asthma treatments as a child. Although he became a strong, energetic adult, he was a sickly child. His bouts of asthma played an important role in the life of his family, who changed their plans many times because of the boy's asthma attacks. No one really knew how to help people with asthma when Teddy Roosevelt was young, but his parents tried anything that they thought would help.

When young Teddy Roosevelt felt the tightening in his chest and began the hacking cough that signaled an asthma attack, it was usually nighttime. He would begin to pant for air. (The word *asthma* is Greek for panting.) Then a high-pitched wheeze would develop. Sitting up helped some, but when he tried to speak, he could say only a few words at a time. He would put his elbows on his knees and battle for breath, gulping for air. All during the attack, he could never get enough air.

On some nights when Teddy suffered from se-

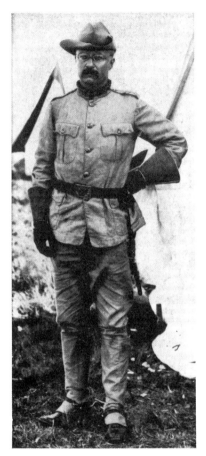

Teddy Roosevelt survived odd treatments for asthma in his childhood, and went on to fight in the Spanish-American War in 1898 (above) and become president in 1901. (Courtesy of the New York Public Library Picture Collection)

vere attacks, his father carried the boy in his arms for hours. Sometimes the servants would be summoned to prepare the carriage for a drive in the outside air, where it was hoped that Teddy would get some relief. Sometimes, this did seem to help.

In his diary, Teddy tells about one night when he sat up for four hours without lying back down on the bed. During that night and on many others, his father made him smoke a cigar. Since we now know that smoking is a trigger for asthma, a cigar seems a strange medicine. One doctor, Henry Hyde Salter, published the book *On Asthma,* in which he tried to explain the purpose of the cigar treatment. He noted that there was no tolerance for tobacco in children, and its use was followed by nausea and vomiting. Dr. Salter wrote that the moment such a condition was present, the asthma ceased. Today there are better ways of stopping an asthma attack.

Coffee was another common medicine for the treatment of asthma in Teddy Roosevelt's time, and it might have been a good one. There are chemicals in coffee that are related to some of the drugs used now to treat kids and adults with asthma, but more concentrated forms of these drugs are used by doctors today.

One very strange yet common treatment was the use of a "mustard plaster." Imagine having mustard on your chest instead of on your hot dog. Doctors suggested soaking a cloth in mustard and a small amount of water and placing the resulting "poultice" on a patient's chest and stomach. Perhaps it was believed that the irritation to the skin that was caused by the mustard would help to dilate, or open, the breathing tubes and thus relieve the asthma.

Another old-fashioned remedy for asthma was made with a teaspoonful of powdered alum mixed with a little molasses. Although molasses tastes good, alum does not. The person with asthma drank some of this mixture every five minutes until he or she vomited. The vomiting may have relaxed the air tubes, for in some cases this treatment did help.

A popular remedy that also induced vomiting was the swallowing of a small amount of ipecac, a medicine that is used today when a child swallows poison and needs to throw up to get rid of it. This, and other treatments that caused vomiting, may have stopped asthma attacks, but they did not relieve the inflammation of the air passages.

More than 2,000 years ago, the Chinese treated asthma with ephedrine, a substance found in some plants. This drug was introduced into Western medicine in 1924 and was used to treat colds and allergies. In recent times, it has been given orally for the treatment of asthma because it relaxes the airways and dries up mucus. However, it causes undesirable side effects such as shakiness and an increase in blood pressure and heart rate. Better asthma medicines have replaced ephedrine.

More recently, injections of gold were a popular treatment for asthma, as well as for tuberculosis and arthritis. Gold does not cure TB or asthma, but it is used to treat one form of arthritis.

Parents tried all sorts of treatments in their efforts to help their children when they were gasping for breath during asthma attacks. Some boys and girls were given enemas. Others were dunked in cold water in an effort to make breathing easier. Some children and adults were made to sniff the fumes of papers treated with certain chemicals. Breathing the awful-smelling smoke of the dried leaves of the jimsonweed was a treatment that was used in North America for centuries. Cases of poisoning from tea made from its seeds were reported in the United States as long ago as 1676. Jimsonweed contains a powerful substance called belladonna, which relaxes the airways and dries the mucous membranes, but it can also be deadly.

One of the more pleasant treatments was the use of cold medicine containing menthol. In a recent speech to a group of students who were studying about asthma, an elderly lady described the times many years earlier when her father would warm the menthol on a pie plate by putting it in the oven. Then he would bring this to her with a glass tube, called a lamp chimney, over the medicine so she could breathe the fumes through the tube until she felt better.

Diets of parsley and cucumbers, eating the meat of an armadillo (an animal found in the South that has tough, horny skin), and wearing copper bracelets or copper-treated shoe inserts have all been tried in efforts to relieve asthma symptoms. There have been claims that these treatments worked, but no one knows whether they really did. Good thoughts do seem to improve the health of many people, so the attitude of relatives and friends may have been the helping factor.

Over the years, the treatments for asthma have become more sophisticated and effective. Although there is still no cure, many excellent medicines are now available that enable those with asthma to control their condition rather than have it control their lives.

7

Medicines in Use Today

SOME asthma medicines reduce the swelling and twitchiness of the air passages, and others open up, or dilate, narrowed airways by relaxing the muscles in the breathing tubes. This allows the person to breathe more freely. Both kinds of drugs are important for the treatment of asthma—the *anti-inflammatory drugs* that reduce swelling and the *bronchodilators* that open up the airways.

A bronchodilator drug called theophylline was widely used for asthma for more than thirty years. It sometimes causes sleeplessness and behavioral problems in children. At high doses, it can cause dangerous reactions such as irregular heartbeat and seizures. Theophylline is still used in some cases, but now there are other bronchodilator medicines available that are more powerful and quicker acting. They fall into a group of drugs known by the long name of *beta-adrenergic agonists* or beta-agonists. Proventil, Brethaire, and Serevent are the trade names of a few that are commonly used. They are man-made relatives of the natural hormone adrenaline. These drugs can be given by mouth or by inhaler. Some are long-acting, lasting 12 hours or more after a single dose, and others have a short duration of action.

Some researchers have linked the continuous use of the beta-adrenergic drugs to the worldwide increases in deaths from asthma. The problem may be the overuse of these medicines and the under-use of medicines that relieve the inflammation of the airways. This is what happened to twenty-year-old football player Mike Ivey, whom we met earlier. He kept inhaling his bronchodilator medicine more and more frequently. This seemed to help for a while because it opened up his airways, but he did not realize that there was a reason why he needed the bronchodilator more and more: His airways were becoming more inflamed, swollen, and clogged with mucus. Bronchodilators could not help that problem, so he was not able to draw enough air into his lungs through the clogged breathing passages.

Doctors emphasize the importance of treating the main problem in asthma, which is the inflammation of the airways. For this they prescribe anti-inflammatory medicines.

The most powerful anti-inflammatory medicines are the *corticosteroids*. Azmacort and Vanceril are two of the brand names of these drugs. They reduce swelling, inflammation, and mucus secretion in severe episodes. In addition, they decrease the sensitivity of the airways in people with allergies. These steroids are not the same as the steroids that are misused by athletes who want to boost their performance.

Corticosteroids taken by mouth or injection are extremely potent drugs that can cause serious side effects when they are used over a long period of time. These side effects include thinning of the bones, increase in blood pressure, ulcers, weakening of the immune system, elevated blood sugar, and slowed growth in children.

Sometimes, when an asthma flare is severe, brief treatment (usually three to five days) with corticosteroids taken by mouth is necessary. When the drugs are used properly, however, they are safe. People should not worry in these situations; used over a period of less than two weeks these steroids do not cause dangerous side effects. It is more important to reduce the inflammation and get the asthma under control.

A major breakthrough in the treatment of asthma has been the development of corticosteroids that can be inhaled, rather than injected or taken by mouth. They are safe when used properly, because they go only to the airways, and are not absorbed into the body. Although there have been some reports of slowed growth in children who used inhaled steroids, most of the children studied showed no negative effects. However, doctors make sure to carefully monitor the growth of children who take steroids over a long period of time.

Other anti-inflammatory drugs are *cromolyn* and a more recent medication called *nedocromil* (Tilade). These drugs cause no adverse side effects. As with inhaled steroids, they are taken by inhaler daily. They may also be used occasionally as a preventive before exercise or before unavoidable exposure to a known allergen.

The newest weapons against asthma are *antileukotrienes.* Leukotrienes are substances that are released from various cells in the body, and they contribute to the inflammation and swelling of the airways during an asthmatic attack. Singulair and other medicines in this group block the action of the leukotrienes. They are used as an alternative to low doses of inhaled steroids or cromolyn or nedocromil for individuals over the age of twelve years who have mild persistent asthma. They have also been approved at lower doses for use by children over age two. Although the antileukotrienes have not caused any bad side effects, experts are monitoring their use carefully because they are new.

Drugs for treating asthma may be *long-term-control medications* that are taken every day in order to control symptoms. These are also known as preventive, controller, or maintenance medications. Or the drugs may be *quick-relief medications,* also called acute rescue medications, that act rapidly to open airways that are severely blocked during an acute attack.

Long-term-control medicines are taken daily to

control persistent asthma. Experts recommend anti-inflammatory drugs such as inhaled steroids or cromolyn to prevent inflammation, and a long-acting bronchodilator drug—a beta-agonist or theophylline. Anti-leukotrienes are also long-term-control drugs. The specific medicines and the dosage vary from individual to individual, depending on whether the asthma is severe or mild, or if an attack occurs only occasionally.

Quick-relief medicines are needed to provide immediate treatment in case of a severe attack. A short-acting beta-agonist, such as Proventil or Brethaire, is given by inhaler, working within 30 minutes to open the narrowed airways. Sometimes oral steroids are given to help speed recovery.

Many people ask about alternative treatments for asthma, such as acupuncture or herbal medicines. Some of these herbal remedies may contain powerful unidentified substances, but so far, none have been proven effective in treating asthma.

Despite the many advances in understanding and treating asthma, there is still concern about the large numbers of children who develop asthma each year. Doctors must find the combination of medicines that is right for each individual. Everyone with asthma should have a written plan for daily treatment and clear instructions about what to do if symptoms worsen or in case of a sudden, severe attack. Children with asthma and their parents can improve their treatment by becoming better educated.

ASTHMA MEDICINES AND THEIR ACTION

BᴿᴼNᴄHᴼᴰIᴸᴬᵀᴼᴿS *(Open the airways)*

▾ Beta-adrenergic agonists (Proventil, Brethaire, Serevent)

> Related to adrenaline but produce fewer side effects. Most powerful medicines for relaxing airways and preventing exercise-induced attacks.

▾ Theophylline (Aerolate)

Aɴᴛɪ-ɪɴꜰʟᴀᴍᴍᴀᴛᴏʀʏ Mᴇᴅɪᴄɪɴᴇꜱ *(Reduce inflammation)*

▾ Corticosteroids (Azmacort, Vanceril)

> Most powerful drugs for reducing inflammation.

▾ Cromolyn and nedocromil (Intal, Tilade)

> May be used instead of corticosteroids as first choice for treating children.
> Also may be used before exercise or before unavoidable exposure to a known allergen.

▾ Anti-leukotrienes (Singulair)

> New drugs used as an alternative to steroids and cromolyn or nedocromil for individuals over the age of 12 years and at a lower dose for children over age two.

Lᴏɴɢ-ᴛᴇʀᴍ-Cᴏɴᴛʀᴏʟ Mᴇᴅɪᴄᴀᴛɪᴏɴꜱ *(Taken daily over a long period of time to control persistent asthma)*

▾ Corticosteroids
▾ Cromolyn and nedocromil
▾ Long-acting beta-agonists (Serevent)
▾ Anti-leukotriene drugs

Qᴜɪᴄᴋ-ʀᴇʟɪᴇꜰ ᴏʀ Rᴇꜱᴄᴜᴇ Mᴇᴅɪᴄᴀᴛɪᴏɴꜱ *(Provide prompt relief for wheezing, coughing, and difficulty breathing by opening narrowed airways)*

▾ Short-acting beta-agonists (Proventil, Brethaire)
▾ Corticosteroids—inhaled or oral

8

Managing Asthma at Home and at School

IF you have asthma, you probably know a lot about how air gets into your lungs when everything is working as it should, and you know what happens when something triggers an attack. You have trouble breathing because your airways become narrowed, swollen, and full of mucus. You probably know what triggers your attacks and what medicines you are supposed to take.

But there is more to managing asthma than going home with a prescription and waiting for the next flare. Too many kids end up in the emergency room every time they have a problem because they are not taking the right medicine or they don't recognize the signs of trouble.

How can you keep your asthma under control? The best way to begin is to find a doctor who is an expert in treating asthma. He or she should take the time to make sure you and your parents have a plan that works for you. It should be a written plan that tells exactly what to do as soon as a problem begins. The plan should say when to take more of one medicine or if you should add another one. The aim is to stop the flare before it gets out of control. When a flare is treated early, less medicine is needed.

The earliest clues of a flare may not be very noticeable. Babies and very young children are not able to say how they feel, but they may act cranky, overactive, upset, or tired. Some kids get itchy around their neck or nose.

Many mothers can predict a flare just by looking at a child's face. Sally's mother—whom we met earlier—learned that dark circles under her daughter's eyes and puffy cheeks meant "asthma alert." If you have a younger brother or sister with asthma, perhaps you have learned to recognize some special warning signs.

Kids with asthma and their families should know the four major trouble signals. If someone with asthma starts to wheeze, breathes faster than normal, breathes out more slowly than in, or sucks in the skin between the ribs when breathing, it means that person needs help.

Kids and adults often do not realize that they are not breathing normally. Of twenty-two people who were recovering in a hospital after being treated for asthma attacks, all thought they were back to

Trouble Signs

- ▾ Wheezing
- ▾ Breathing faster than normal
- ▾ Breathing out more slowly than breathing in
- ▾ Sucking in of chest skin

normal again. But tests showed that none of them were breathing normally.

If you have asthma, you should know that even before you begin to wheeze, your airways have already started to get narrower. In fact, by the time a doctor can hear any changes in your lungs with a stethoscope, the ability to push air out of your lungs has already dropped 25 percent. For this reason, asthma experts think that it is important for people with asthma to use a very simple device called a *peak flow meter* (pictured on p. 57). This instrument measures the amount of air that a person can blow out quickly. It is both safe and easy to use.

Peter's doctor tested his breathing with a peak flow meter when he had his first asthma attack at age seven. The nurse helped Peter and his mother practice using it correctly so they could do the same thing at home. First, they set the indicator at zero. Peter took the chewing gum out of his mouth and stood up. He took a slow, deep breath with his

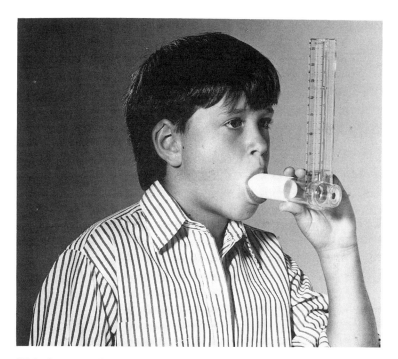

This boy uses his peak flow meter to measure how much air he can blow out of his lungs. (Courtesy of Fisons Corporation)

mouth open and took in as much air as he could. Then he put the mouthpiece in his mouth, and he blew out as hard and as fast as he could. The force of the air pushed the pointer up the numbered scale. The number that the pointer indicated (called the *peak expiratory flow rate*) showed how much air he was able to blow out of his lungs in one fast huff. Peter repeated this procedure two more times, and the nurse recorded the highest number, which indicated his best try out of three.

There are charts that show the average peak flow

rates for your height and sex. But everyone is different. If you have asthma, it is important to find out
what your own normal peak flow is when you are
feeling good. Peter's doctor asked his mother to
check his peak flow at home three times a day and
keep a record of his best tries, so they would know
his normal measurement.

The peak flow measurements fall into three
zones: green, yellow, and red. The green zone is 80
to 100 percent of your personal best. This is the
healthy zone. The yellow zone is 50 to 80 percent
of your normal peak flow number, and it means
that your lung function is reduced. Even if you do
not notice any difficulty breathing, this is the cau-
tion zone. In the yellow zone, you are more sensitive to triggers, and a flare may be set off very
quickly. If your measurements fall into the red
zone (less than 50 percent of your peak flow), you
are in real danger and need treatment quickly.

The peak flow meter is the best tool for keeping
track of asthma treatment at home because it re-
moves a lot of guesswork about what is really happening in your lungs. It means that treatment can
be started early, when it is needed to ward off an
attack. It can also warn kids and families when
there is a serious emergency. Knowing peak flow is
a good way to tell if your medicines are working.

Some children do not like to admit that they are
having symptoms of a flare. They may not want
their friends to think they are weak or sickly, so

they ignore the warning signs and get into trouble. The peak flow meter lets parents know before more serious trouble begins. By contrast, other children may exaggerate their breathing problems and use asthma as an excuse for not participating in activities. The peak flow meter helps parents determine what's really going on.

Whereas using the peak flow meter enables you to measure the amount of air your lungs can expel, practicing a variety of breathing exercises can serve to strengthen and expand this capability. Breathing exercises can help anyone get through an asthma attack, participate in sports, and enjoy a more normal life. (Of course, they are no substitute for medicine.)

Here are some breathing exercises you can try:

There is a large muscle in your body known as the diaphragm. It is beneath your lungs and above your abdomen (stomach area). The diaphragm moves up and down as you breathe. By concentrating on it, you can learn to breathe so that you use your lungs more fully. Most people do not use their lungs fully when they breathe, for they get enough air without doing so. People with asthma, however, can benefit by learning to use their whole lung capacity.

Breathe in through your nose, counting as you do so. Hold your hand on your abdomen and notice how it extends as you breathe in. Now breathe out, counting to yourself for twice as long as you did when you breathed in. Keep your hand over the upper part of your abdomen and pull in the muscles as you breathe out. Repeat this exercise three times.

Another breathing exercise that is popular among people who want to relax is done sitting in a chair. You lean forward, while keeping your back straight. You put your arms on your knees. This makes your shoulders drop. Hold your lips in a whistling position. Then breathe in through your nose and breathe out slowly through your mouth without moving your chest. Do this for a few minutes.

Blowing up balloons and practicing on a musical instrument such as a trumpet, clarinet, and flute can also help to increase your lung power.

Managing asthma at school can be a challenge. Amy's experiences illustrate some of the problems involved.

Eight-year-old Amy takes her asthma medicine regularly, and she is careful to avoid petting cats because she's allergic to cat dander. She is also allergic to ragweed, so in the fall she has to be more careful about watching for the signs of a flare. She knows when she may have trouble because her chest starts feeling tight. If she uses her inhaler immediately, she can stop the attack. If she doesn't, she gets worse very quickly and sometimes ends up in the hospital.

Amy knows how and when to use the inhaler and is very conscientious. She always carries her inhaler when she goes out to play or when she goes someplace with her parents. But at school, where she is a third-grader, she cannot keep her inhaler with her.

As in many other places throughout the country, the state where Amy lives has a rule that does not allow students to keep any medicine with them. The school nurse must keep her inhaler. This means that when Amy feels the warnings of a flare, she has to ask the teacher to excuse her from class, and she must go to the nurse's office. If the nurse is busy taking care of an emergency with another child, Amy has to wait. Sometimes she has been delayed for as long as thirty minutes. During that time, her breathing got worse. In addition, she does not like missing time in class. She also feels embarrassed about calling attention to herself by asking to be excused. She does not want her classmates to think she is a sick person.

Amy's mother and a lot of other people think that children with asthma should be allowed to carry their inhalers with them at all times, so they can stop a flare without delay. But school officials say they have rules about medicine because they are afraid that children might not know how much to take and might endanger themselves without the help of a nurse. They are also afraid that other children would want to experiment with an inhaler that belongs to a child with asthma.

One nurse who works at a middle school in an inner-city neighborhood says that many of the fifty children with asthma who attend that school do not know what medicines they are on and do not know anything about asthma. She worries that they might use their inhalers improperly or even lose them. They might have a serious attack without her knowing about it.

But Nancy Sander, mother of a child with asthma and founder of a group called the National Allergy and Asthma Network, says that making children go to the nurse's office for their inhalers is like making them go there to get their eyeglasses or hearing aids.

Occasionally, someone does take too much medicine. For instance, a high school hockey player overuses his inhaler so he does not have to stop playing in the middle of a game. But most children use their inhalers responsibly. Even if someone else tried to use the inhaler, it probably would not cause any harm.

Some doctors think that junior and senior high school students should be allowed to take care of their own medicine if the kid's parents and doctor give their approval. Some younger children are not old enough or mature enough, but many are, as in Amy's case.

If you have asthma, it is very important for your

teacher and school nurse to be informed about your condition so they will know what to do if you have a problem. This means that your parents and doctor need to give the school your medicines and instructions about what to do in case you have a flare.

Sometimes problems come up when a gym teacher does not know that asthma flares can be triggered by exercise. This teacher thinks that the student is trying to avoid gym because he or she is lazy. It is important for the doctor to write a letter explaining what exercise-induced asthma is and how it can be controlled. The letter should also explain that cold air might trigger an attack when a kid with asthma goes outside to play during recess. The classroom teacher should know that a class pet can trigger a flare in someone who is allergic to the animal.

Some asthma medicines cause side effects such as overactivity. A kid might act fidgety and misbehave as a result of the medicine, not because he or she is bad. You can see why it is important for the teacher to know that someone is taking medicine that could have this kind of unwanted effect.

Even if you have asthma, you can probably do just about anything that everyone else is doing, as long as you know how to keep your special problems in check. You can control asthma by using a peak flow meter, practicing breathing exercises, recognizing and avoiding triggers, knowing trouble signs, using medicine properly, and following your doctor's treatment plan. You *can* stay healthy most of the time. And you do not need to consider yourself sick or different from your friends and classmates.

9

Sports and Camps for Kids with Asthma

IN twenty minutes, a team of swimmers is going to race. One of them has had asthma all her life, but she is a winner in almost every race. Now she takes two puffs from her inhaler, puts on her suit, tucks her hair under her racing cap, and lines up with the team. She can really pour on the speed when she enters the pool, for the medicine relaxes her airways and prevents an asthma flare. While she is racing, her asthma is on the back burner and swimming is the most important thing in her life.

From 60 to 90 percent of people with asthma suffer an attack when exercise is strenuous over a long period of time. Symptoms do not usually appear until five or ten minutes after exercise. Scientists think that the loss of heat and water from cells in the airways during exercise plays a part in causing an attack.

Sometimes kids with asthma think they are people who were not made for sports. However, many of them learn that they can enjoy sports and feel better because they exercise. One man, who is now a doctor, had asthma from the age of three. Now he is forty-nine years old and still has asthma, but he changed from a person who was afraid to participate in sports to one who runs daily. He has run in the New York and Boston marathons and says that running "overcomes his asthma." He runs with an inhaler clenched in his hand, but he feels that his asthma gets worse when he does not run.

Nancy Hogshead used to pass out repeatedly as a teenager after swim practice and races until she learned that she had exercise-induced asthma. She received treatment to control her asthma and became an Olympic swimmer. She earned three gold medals at the 1984 Olympic Games.

In her book *Asthma and Exercise,* Nancy describes the experiences of many famous athletes who have this condition. She describes how asthma affected her life, too. She does not think that she wastes much energy keeping her asthma under control, for she is so busy with swimming that asthma control is routine. She likes to compare controlling her asthma with what she does to keep her teeth clean and healthy. Every day, she flosses and brushes her teeth. She sees her dentist twice a year and makes an extra visit if there is a special problem. Her daily routine to keep her teeth healthy is not something she thinks about very much. The same is true in the case of her asthma control program. She uses her inhaler and her peak flow meter, and records her exposure to triggers as part of her daily routine. These actions are as automatic as brushing her teeth.

One of the most famous athletes with asthma is Jackie Joyner-Kersee. This 1988 double gold medalist is considered by many experts to be the top female track-and-field athlete in the world. She used to dislike taking medicine, but she found out how important it was to follow her doctor's orders one day when she was training. The day was cold, and the grass in the stadium had just been mowed. This combination was enough to trigger a serious asthma attack. As she reached the top step in the stadium, Jackie knew something was wrong. She couldn't breathe, and she felt hot. She bent over, trying to catch her breath, and she started to panic. Even a few puffs with her inhaler did not stop the attack. Her husband, who was also her coach, rushed her to the hospital where she was treated in the emergency room. Later, through blood tests, Jackie's doctor found that she was not taking her medicine properly.

Jackie says that she really felt as if she was going to die before she was successfully treated in the emergency room. Now she takes her pills and uses her inhaler regularly in the program recommended by her doctor.

The list of famous athletes with asthma is long, but not every kid with asthma can, or wants to, become a serious athlete. Nevertheless, many kids who regard themselves as "klutzy" because they think they cannot handle any kind of physical exertion learn to have fun with sports and dancing. Some of them learn to enjoy more physical activities and keep their asthma in check by attending asthma camps for a week or two.

Spending a week or two at a special camp for kids with asthma is becoming more popular than ever. Camp Treasure Chest in Chester, Connecticut, is typical. It offers water sports, arts, crafts, campfire sessions, and additional activities that are found at many other camps, but there are some activities that are different. These are Treasure Chest sessions in which kids learn about asthma, for every camper has this condition.

Camp Treasure Chest is one of thirty to forty camps throughout the United States that are especially designed for kids with asthma. Asthma camps have round-the-clock medical supervision, with many staff members volunteering their services. They have wonderful names such as: Camp Superkids, Camp Not-A-Wheeze, Champ Camp, Camp Superstuff, Sunshine Station Camp, Camp Huff and Puff. If you are interested in finding an asthma camp near you, contact the American Lung Association in your area.

One of the special benefits of going to an asthma

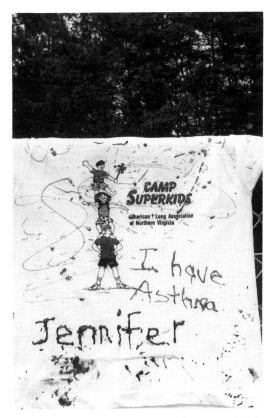

At an asthma camp, learning about asthma can be fun. (Courtesy of the American Lung Association)

camp is learning to participate in sports that seemed out of reach. The camper also learns to feel like a person who happens to have asthma rather than an "asthmatic." He or she improves asthma management skills and so feels more confident and independent—not just at camp but all year long.

Most kids with asthma do not attend these special camps. They need guidance when it comes to deciding which types of exercise to engage in and taking steps to minimize the health risks posed by exercise. Here is some advice for those of you with asthma who are considering your exercise options:

It's a good idea to choose a sport that does not keep you in action for long periods, such as baseball, soccer, football, weightlifting, golf, or swimming. Team sports that require short bursts of energy are good sports for kids with asthma. However, many people with asthma are outstanding runners and basketball players. A careful plan allows most people with asthma to participate in almost any kind of exercise.

Try to avoid exercises that take place in cold, dry places. But if you do decide to take up ice-skating or cross-country skiing, use a face mask or scarf over your nose to warm and moisten the air you breathe. With help from doctors and trainers, some athletes with asthma have become excellent skiers. Bill Koch became a world champion cross-country skier.

Swimming is considered to be the best sport for a person with exercise-induced asthma because the swimmer breathes warm, moist air as he or she exercises. Some doctors recommend that people with asthma choose swimming as their sport. Other doctors maintain that the individual—not the doctor—

should be the one to choose the activity he or she enjoys the most. They believe that everyone with well-controlled asthma can participate in every sport.

If you have asthma and enjoy swimming, you may be tempted to try scuba diving. But this can be dangerous for people with asthma. The cold water, the dry air that is breathed through the mask, and the physical exertion can all act as triggers for an asthma attack, which could result in drowning. Another danger can occur when a diver rises toward the surface, since the air in the lungs expands then. The person with asthma who is having trouble exhaling may have such a large amount of air trapped in the lungs that it can damage or even rupture the lung tissue as it expands. It is important for people with asthma to know that they should avoid scuba diving.

Warm up with nonstrenuous exercises before you begin your sport and do cool-down exercises afterward.

Check with your doctor about the proper use of your inhaler before exercising. Too frequent use without checking with your doctor about inflammation of airways can be dangerous.

Also ask your doctor for back-up medicine if your asthma flares up and symptoms continue after you stop exercising.

Glossary

Allergen: A protein substance foreign to the body that triggers an allergic reaction in a susceptible person. Ragweed pollen is an allergen that is the major cause of allergy in the United States. Other examples are dust, mold, and animal dander.

Allergy: Reaction (sneezing, congestion, and runny nose, for example) caused by contact with an allergen such as ragweed pollen.

Alveoli: Latin word for the tiny elastic air sacs that make up the lung tissue. (A single air sac is called an alveolus.)

Antibodies: Proteins made by the immune system to protect the body against invaders like bacteria or viruses. In allergy, a special kind of antibody (called IgE) is made against ordinarily harmless substances like food, dust, or pollen. It usually takes at least two years of breathing an allergen like ragweed pollen before the person makes enough antibody to result in allergy symptoms.

Anti-inflammatory medicines: Medicines that reduce inflammation. Cromolyn, nedocromil, anti-leukotrienes, and corticosteroids are used to treat airway inflammation in asthma.

Bacteria: Microscopic one-celled organisms, many of which are responsible for various kinds of disease. Examples are strep throat, tuberculosis, and some types of pneumonia. (Singular form is bacterium.)

Beta-adrenergic agonists: Group of medicines that have an action similar to adrenaline (epinephrine) but with fewer unwanted side effects. Very effective for opening narrowed airways.

Bronchi: Large air tubes that branch off the windpipe. One bronchus goes to each lung.

Bronchioles: Small air tubes that branch off the bronchi and lead to the alveoli.

Bronchodilator: Medicine that opens up or dilates the airways. Adrenaline (epinephrine), theophylline, and beta-adrenergic agonists such as Atrovent and Proventil are some examples of bronchodilators.

Corticosteroids: Powerful medicines that reduce swelling and inflammation. Inhaled forms of these medicines work on asthma but do not produce unwanted side effects.

Dander: Tiny particles of skin, hair, or feathers that can float in the air. When they are breathed in, they may cause an allergic reaction.

Emphysema: Damage or destruction of the walls of

the air sacs, leading to interference with the exchange of oxygen and carbon dioxide in the lungs. The most common cause is cigarette smoking. Emphysema is *not* caused by asthma.

Epinephrine: See adrenaline.

Flare: Asthma attack. Onset of symptoms such as tightness in the chest, a dry, hacking cough, coughing up mucus, wheezing, shortness of breath, or trouble exhaling.

Inflammation: Reaction of body tissues—for instance, to injury or allergy—that causes an accumulation of fluid and white blood cells and enlargement of blood vessels in the area. If you fall and scrape your knee, you may notice oozing of fluid from the scraped skin and your knee may become swollen. The fluid contains white blood cells, some of which fight infection. In asthma, the lining of the airways becomes swollen and thickened because of the fluid and white blood cells that have oozed out of the blood vessels. This swelling results in a narrowing of the airways and interferes with breathing.

Inhaler: Device that delivers medicine in vaporized form that can be breathed in.

Mast cells: Allergy-causing cells. Found throughout the body but very numerous in tissues that line the nose and lungs. The allergy-causing antibodies (IgE) sit on the mast cells, and when an allergen like ragweed pollen is inhaled, it triggers the mast cells to release chemicals that cause the symptoms of allergy. These chemicals are also the cause of the airway problems in asthma.

Mucus: Secretion normally made by cells in the nose and airways. It protects against infection and keeps the tissues from drying out. It increases and becomes sticky during an asthma attack and can plug up the airways.

Peak flow meter: Device you blow into that measures how well your airways are working. Its use is a good way of monitoring asthma.

Status asthmaticus: Term used to describe severe asthma symptoms that do not respond to the usual treatment. It is a life-threatening condition if not treated vigorously.

Sulfites: Chemicals used as preservatives in some foods, wines, beer, and medicines. Can cause asthma attacks in some people.

Trachea: Windpipe. Air breathed in through the nose and mouth goes through the trachea into the bronchi, then through the bronchioles to the air sacs in the lungs.

Triggers: Conditions that set off an asthma attack, such as allergy, exercise, cold, or infection.

Twitchiness: Term used to describe the overreactivity of the airways in people with asthma. Twitchy airways are supersensitive and react to triggers such as allergens, cold, exercise, and infections by tightening the tiny muscles in their walls and causing narrowing of the breathing tubes.

Virus: The tiniest of organisms, smaller than bacteria, a packet of molecules made up of a core of genetic material with an outer coat of protein. Dependent on bacteria, plant, or animal cells and cannot live on its own. Hundreds of different viruses are responsible for disease in people. Colds, measles, polio, hepatitis, and AIDS are all caused by viruses.

Wheezing: Whistling sound, usually associated with difficulty in breathing caused by constricted airways, as in asthma. Wheezing may be caused by conditions other than asthma and is not always present in asthma.

For Further Information

American Lung Association
www.lungusa.com
Check your phone book for the chapter nearest you.

Asthma and Allergy Foundation of America
11233 20th Street, NW
Suite 402
Washington, DC 20036
1-800-7-ASTHMA (800-727-8462)
www.aafa.org
Hotline for questions about medicines, referrals, camps.

Allergy and Asthma Network • Mothers of
  Asthmatics, Inc.
2751 Prosperity Avenue, Suite 150
Fairfax, VA 22031
1-800-878-4403
www.aanma.org
*Issues a newsletter eight times a year and a magazine four
  times a year.*

National Institutes of Health
9000 Rockville Pike
Bethesda, MD 20892
301-496-4000
Ask for information on asthma.

National Jewish Medical and Research Center
1400 Jackson Street
Denver, CO 80206
1-800-222-LUNG (in Denver: 355-LUNG)
*Hotline for questions about asthma and other lung
diseases.*

OTHER HELPFUL WEBSITES
www.thriveonline.com/health/asthma/
Useful tools for kids, teens, and parents.

www.healthanswers.com/
Information on symptoms and medications.

Suggestions for Further Reading

Hogshead, Nancy, and Gerald S. Couzens. *Asthma and Exercise*. New York: Henry Holt, 1989.

Kerby, Mona. *Asthma*. New York: Franklin Watts, 1989.

Ostrow, William, and Vivian Ostrow. *All About Asthma*. Morton Grove, Ill.: Albert Whitman, 1989.

Rogers, Alison. *Luke Has Asthma, Too*. Burlington, Vt.: Waterfront Books, 1987.

Sander, Nancy. *I'm A Meter Reader*. Research Triangle Park, N.C.: Allen and Hanburys, Glaxo, 1990. (For very young children.)

Sander, Nancy. *So You Have Asthma Too!* Research Triangle Park, N.C.: Allen and Hanburys, 1991. (For very young children.)

Spector, Sheldon, and Nancy Sander. *Understanding Asthma: A Blueprint For Breathing*. Palatine, Ill.: American College of Allergy and Immunology, 3rd ed., 1991.

Index